AIR FRYER COOKBOOK

FISH AND SEAFOOD

RECIPES

Quick, Easy and Delicious Recipes for healthy living while keeping your weight under control

Nancy Johnson

Copyright © 2021 by Nancy Johnson

Legal Disclaimer

The information contained in this book and its contents is not designed to replace any form of medical or professional advice; and is not meant to replace the need for independent medical, financial, legal, or other professional advice or service that may require. The content and information in this book have been provided for educational and entertainment purposes only.

The content and information contained in this book have been compiled from sources deemed reliable, and they are accurate to the best of the Author's knowledge, information and belief.

However, the Author cannot guarantee its accuracy and validity and therefore cannot be held liable for any errors and/or omissions.

Further, changes are periodically made to this book as needed. Where appropriate and/or necessary, you must consult a professional (including but not limited to your doctor, attorney, financial advisor, or other such professional) before using any of the suggested remedies, techniques, and/or information in this book.

Upon using this book's contents and information, you agree to hold harmless the Author from any damaged, costs and expenses, including any legal fees potentially resulting from the application of any of the information in this book. This disclaimer applies to any loss, damages, or injury caused by the use and application of this book's content, whether directly and indirectly, whether for breach of contract, tort, negligence, personal injury, criminal intent, or under any other circumstances.

You agree to accept all risks of using the information presented in this book. You agree that by continuing to read this book, where appropriate and/or necessary, you shall consult a professional (including but not limited to your doctor, attorney, financial advisor, or other such professional) before remedies, techniques, and/or information in this book.

TABLE OF CONTENTS

1. Yummy Pollock 8

2. Honey Sea Bass.. 10

3. Tilapia Sauce and Chives 12

4. Tilapia Coconut.. 13

5. Catfish Fillets Special 15

6. Tasty French Cod 17

7. Oriental Fish... 19

8. Salmon with Blackberry Glaze 21

9. Swiss Chard and Lemon Sole 23

10. Branzino Air Fried... 25

11. Snapper Vegetables and Fillets 27

12. Tasty Red Snapper 28

13. Seasoned Salmon.. 30

14. Spanish Salmon 31

15. Unique Lettuce... 33

16. Salmon Sauce and Greek Yogurt....................... 35

17. Salmon and Avocado Meal 37

18. Hawaiian Lettuce.. 39

19. Cod and Pearl Onions....................................... 40

20. Chinese Cod 41

21. Marine and Seafish 42

22. Black Cod and Plum Sauce................................ 44

23. Sun-Dried Tomatoes and Halibut Blend 46

24. Prosciutto and Grilled Cod.................................48

25. Vinaigrette Salmon with Chives 49

26. Stuffed Calamari 50

27. Beaked Salmon..52

28. Salmon and Sauce with Avocado........................53

29. Lemon and Fish Relish..55

30. Chili Salmon 57

31. Marmalade of Savory and Orange 59

32. Swordfish, with Salsa Mango 60

33. Thai Fish Cakes AirFryer Style 62

34. Aromatized Jamaican Salmon 64

35. Mustard Salmon 66

36. Flaked Salmon 67

37. Shrimp and Cauliflower 69

38. Squid and Guacamole 71

39. Chimichurri and Fish Sauce 73

40. Creamy Vegetables and Shrimp 75

41. Italian Tomato Salsa and Barramundi Filets 77

42. Salsa with Salmon and Avocado.........................79

43. Creamy Salmon 81

44. Trout and Sauce with Butter..............................82

45. Thyme and Parsley Salmon 83

46. Fillet Cod and Peas 84

47. Fillet Truffle and Orange Sauce.........................86

48. Casserole Seafood 87

49. Shrimp and Mix with Crab.................................89

50. Cod and Vinaigrette 91

51. Asian Halibut 93

52. Marine Lemon Saba 95

53. Salmon with Capers and Mash 96

54. Aromatized Air Fried Salmon 98

55. Steaks Cod with Plum Sauce 100

56. Asian Salmon... 101

57. Buttered Shrimp Skewers 102

58. Shrimp Tabasco 103

59. Cod Cutlets with Salad Fennel and Grapes.......... 105

60. Tasty Catfish 107

AIR FRYER COOKBOOK: FISH AND SEAFOOD RECIPES

1. Yummy Pollock

Prep Time about 25 min | Servings 6 | Normal

INGREDIENTS:

- 1/2 cup of sour cream
- 4 Pollock fillets, barefoot
- 1/4 cup Parmesan, rubbed
- 2 tablespoons of sugar, melted
- Salt and black chili, to the taste
- Cooking spray

DIRECTIONS:

1. Mix the sour cream in a dish of butter, parmesan, salt, and pepper and whisk fine.

2. Sprinkle fish with spray to fry and season with salt and pepper.

3. Place the sour cream mixture on each side of Pollock fillet, arrange in hot AirFryer oven at 320° F, then cook for 15 minutes.

4. Divide Pollock fillets into bowls, and serve with a delightful side salad.

Enjoy!

Nutrition: Calories: 300, Fat: 13 g, Fiber: 3 g, Carbohydrates: 14 g, Protein: 44 g.

2. Honey Sea Bass

Prep Time about 20 min | Servings 2 | Normal

INGREDIENTS:

- ➢ 2 fillets of sea bass
- ➢ 1/2 orange zest, rubbed
- ➢ 1/2 fruit juice
- ➢ 1 tablespoon of black pepper and salt
- ➢ 2 mustard spoons
- ➢ 2 honey teaspoons
- ➢ 2 pounds of olive oil
- ➢ 1/2 pound of dried, drained lentils
- ➢ A tiny amount of dill, chopped
- ➢ 2 ounces of cress water
- ➢ A tiny amount of chopped parsley

DIRECTIONS:

1. Add salt and peppered fish fillets, apply citrus zest and juice, rub with 1 spoonful of milk, honey, and mustard, and pass to your Air Fry and cook for 10 minutes at 350° F, turning in half.

2. In the meantime, place the lentils in a small pot, heat them up over medium heat, add the milk, watercress, dill and parsley, mix well and split between plates.

3. Insert the fish fillets and serve promptly.

Enjoy it!

Nutrition: Calories: 212, Fat: 8g, Fiber: 12 g, Carbohydrates: 9 g, Protein: 17 g.

3. Tilapia Sauce and Chives

Prep Time about 18 min | Servings 4 | Normal

INGREDIENTS:

➢ 4 Medium fillets with tilapia

➢ Cooking spray

➢ Salt and black chili, to taste

➢ 2 teaspoons honey

➢ 1/4 cup Greek yogurt

➢ 1 lemon juice

➢ 2 spoonful of chives, chopped

DIRECTIONS:

1. Season with salt and pepper, sprinkle with mist, put in hot oven 350° F AirFryer and cook for ten minutes, tossing midway.

2. In the meantime, blend yogurt with sugar, salt, vinegar, vinegar, and chives in a cup, whisk lemon juice.

3. Divide AirFryer fish into bowls, chop yogurt sauce and serve immediately.

Enjoy!

Nutrition: Calories: 261, Fat: 8 g, Fiber: 18 g, Carbohydrates: 24 g, Protein: 21 g.

4. Tilapia Coconut

Prep Time about 20 min | Servings 4 | Normal

INGREDIENTS:

➢ 4 medium fillets with tilapia

➢ Salt and black chili, to taste

➢ 1/2 cup of cocoon milk

➢ 1 ginger-spoon, rubbed

➢ 1/2 cup of cilantro

➢ 2 sliced cloves of garlic

➢ 1/2 teaspoon of garam masala

➢ Cooking spray

➢ Half jalapeno, split

DIRECTIONS:

1. Mix the coconut milk with salt, pepper, cilantro in your food processor, ginger, garlic, jalapeno, with garam masala, and always pulse well.

2. Sprinkle fish with cooking oil, scatter coconut mixes around, rub well. Switch to the basket with the AirFryer and cook at 400° F for 10 minutes.

3. Divide between plates and serve hot.

Enjoy!

Nutrition: Calories: 200, Fat: 5 g, Fiber: 6 g, Carbohydrates: 25 g, Protein: 26 g.

5. Catfish Fillets Special

Prep Time about 22 min | Servings 4 | Normal

INGREDIENTS:

➤ 2 catfish fillets

➤ 1/2 teaspoon of ginger

➤ 2 ounces of butter

➤ 4 ounces of Worcestershire sauce

➤ 1/2 cubicle jerk seasoning

➤ 1 mustard casserole

➤ 1 spoonful of balsamic vinegar

➤ 3/4 cup Catsup

➤ Salt and black chili, to taste

➤ 1 spoonful of parsley, chopped

DIRECTIONS:

1. Heat a skillet over medium heat with the butter, add Worcestershire sauce, seasoning, garlic, mustard, catsup, vinegar, salt, and hot pepper. Adjust fire, swirl well, and apply fish fillets.

2. Toss well, leave the fillets for 10 minutes, drain them, pass them to the preheated oven, 350° F AirFryer basket, and cook for 8 minutes halfway through flip fillets.

3. Divide into bowls, brush on top with parsley and serve immediately.

Enjoy!

Nutrition: Calories: 351, Fat: 8 g, Fiber: 16 g, Carbohydrates: 27 g, Protein: 17 g.

6. Tasty French Cod

Prep Time about 32 min | Servings 4 | Normal

INGREDIENTS:

➢ 2 tsp of olive oil

➢ 1 yellow onion, sliced

➢ 1/2 cup White wine

➢ 2 cloves of garlic, minced

➢ 14 ounces of dried, stewed tomatoes

➢ 3 teaspoons of parsley

➢ 2 lbs. of cod, boneless

➢ Salt and black chili, to taste

➢ 2 tablespoons of butter

DIRECTIONS:

1. Heat a saucepan over medium heat with the oil, add garlic and onion, stir, and just cook for five minutes.

2. Insert wine, stir and proceed to cook for 1 minute.

3. Stir in tomatoes, bring to a boil, simmer for 2 minutes, add fuel, and stir. Then turn the sun off again.

4. Form of this combination into a heat-proof dish that suits your fryer, add chicken, season with salt and pepper, and steam 350° F in your fryer for fourteen minutes.

5. Divide the tomatoes and the fish into plates and serve.

Enjoy!

Nutrition: Calories: 231, Fat: 8 g, Fiber: 12 g, Carbohydrates: 26 g, Protein: 14 g.

7. Oriental Fish

Prep Time about 22 min | Servings 4 | Normal

INGREDIENTS:

➢ 2 lbs of red snapper fillets, knobbles

➢ Salt and black chili, to taste

➢ 3 cloves of garlic, minced

➢ 1 yellow onion, sliced

➢ 1 tamarind paste cubic

➢ 1 tablespoon of oriental sesame oil

➢ 1 tsp of ginger, grated

➢ 2 cups of water

➢ 1/2 cumin cubicle, land

➢ 1 tsp of lemon juice

➢ 3 spoons mint, chopped

DIRECTIONS:

1. Mix the garlic with the onion, salt, pepper, and tamarind in your mixing bowl. Add the paste, sesame oil, ginger, cumin, and water, pulse well, and scrub the fish with that combination.

2. Place the fish at 320° F in your preheated AirFryer and cook for 12 minutes halfway, tossing fish.

3. Divide fish over bowls, chop lemon juice, sprinkle mint, and serve immediately.

Enjoy!

Nutrition: Calories: 241, Fat: 8 g, Fiber: 16 g, Carbohydrates: 17 g, Protein: 12 g.

8. Salmon with Blackberry Glaze

Prep Time about 43 min | Servings 4 | Normal

INGREDIENTS:

➢ 1 cup of water

➢ 1 inch of slice of ginger, grated

➢ 1/2 lemon juice

➢ 12 ounces of blackberries

➢ 1 Tsp of olive oil

➢ 1/2 cup of sugar

➢ 4 medium fillets trout, skinless

➢ Salt and black chili, to taste

DIRECTIONS:

1. Heat up a casserole with water over a moderate flame. Add ginger, lemon. Stir in the juice and blackberries, bring to a simmer, simmer for 4-5 minutes, extract in a cup, cover, rinse, return to the pan and mix with the sugar.

2. Bring this mixture to a boil over medium-low heat and simmer for 20 minutes.

3. Leave blackberry sauce to cool, sprinkle with salmon, season with salt and pepper, drizzle all over the olive oil and scrape well.

4. Place the fish at 350° F in your preheated AirFryer and cook for 10 minutes; the fish fillets rotated once.

5. Divide into bowls, add each of the leftover blackberry sauce up and serve.

Enjoy!

Nutrition: Calories: 312, Fat: 4 g, Fiber: 9 g, Carbohydrates: 19 g, Protein: 14 g.

9. Swiss Chard and Lemon Sole

Prep Time about 24 min | Servings 4 | Normal

INGREDIENTS:

➢ 1 tsp of lemon zest

➢ 4 slices of white bread, quartered,

➢ 1/4 cup of walnuts, chopped

➢ Parmesan: 1/4 cup, rubbed

➢ 4 lbs. of olive oil

➢ 4 single, boneless fillets

➢ Salt and black chili, to taste

➢ 4 cups of butter

➢ 1/4 cup of lemon juice

➢ 3 spoons of capers

➢ 2 cloves of garlic, minced

➢ 2 swiss chard bunches, diced

DIRECTIONS:

1. Mix the bread with the walnuts, cheese, and lemon zest in your food processor, and then pulse well.

2. Apply half of the olive oil, pulse again really good, and set for now aside.

3. Warm the butter over a moderate flame on a saucepan, add lemon juice, salt. Stir well, pepper and capers, add the tuna, and toss.

4. Switch the fish to the basket of your hot oven AirFryer, cover with bread mix, and cook for 14 minutes at 350° F.

5. In the meantime, fire up another saucepan with the remaining oil, add garlic, Swiss chard, salt and pepper, stir gently, and simmer for 2 minutes, then turn off.

6. Divide the tuna into plates and serve horizontally with a sautéed chard.

Enjoy it!

Nutrition: Calories: 321, Fat: 7 g, Fiber: 18 g, Carbohydrates: 27 g, Protein: 12 g.

10. Branzino Air Fried

Prep Time about 20 min | Servings 4 | Normal

INGREDIENTS:

- ➢ 1 lemon zest, grated
- ➢ 1 orange zest, grated
- ➢ 1/2 lemon juice
- ➢ 1/2 orange juice
- ➢ Salt and black pepper, to taste
- ➢ 4 medium fillets of branzino, boneless
- ➢ 1/2 cup of parsley
- ➢ 2 Pounds of olive oil
- ➢ A slice of red, ground pepper flakes

DIRECTIONS:

1. Mix the fish fillets in a large bowl with the citrus zest, orange zest, lemon juice, orange juice, salt, pepper, flakes of oil and pepper, swirl well, pass the filets thoroughly at 350° F on your preheated AirFryer and bake for 10 minutes, one fillet tossing once.

2. Splash fish on bowls, scatter with parsley and serve promptly.

Enjoy!

Nutrition: Calories: 261, Fat: 8 g, Fiber: 12 g, Carbohydrates: 21 g, Protein: 12 g.

11. Snapper Vegetables and Fillets

Prep Time about 24 min | Servings 2 | Normal

INGREDIENTS:

➢ 2 red snapper fillets, boneless

➢ 1 tablespoon of olive oil

➢ 1/2 cup of red pepper

➢ 1/2 cup of green pepper

➢ 1/2 cup of leeks, split

➢ Salt and black chili, to taste

➢ 1 tsp, dry tarragon

➢ Sprinkled with white wine

DIRECTIONS:

1. Comb the fish fillets with salt in a heatproof tray that suits your AirFryer. Add pepper, oil, green pepper, red pepper, leeks, tarragon, and wine. Toss all well, install 350° F in preheated AirFryer, and cook, tossing fish fillets halfway, for 14 minutes.

2. Divide fish and veggies into bowls, served wet.

Enjoy!

Nutrition: Calories: 300, Fat: 12 g, Fiber: 8 g, Carbohydrates: 29 g, Protein: 12 g.

12. Tasty Red Snapper

Prep Time about 45 min | Servings 4 | Normal

INGREDIENTS:

- ➢ 1 wide red snapper, tidy and scored
- ➢ Salt and black chili, to taste
- ➢ 3 cloves of garlic, minced
- ➢ 1 jalapeno, split
- ➢ 1/4 lb of okra, hacked
- ➢ 1 tablespoon of butter
- ➢ 2 tablespoon of olive oil
- ➢ 1 chopped red bell pepper
- ➢ 2 Spoonful of white wine
- ➢ 2 Peregrinated spoons, chopped

DIRECTIONS:

1. Mix jalapeno, wine, and garlic in a cup, stir well and fry with a snapper that combination.

2. Season with salt and pepper and put on for 30 minutes.

3. In the meantime, fire up a saucepan over medium heat with 1 tablespoon butter, add mix in pepper and okra, and cook for 5 minutes.

4. Fill the red snapper's belly with this combination, introduce the parsley, and rub with olive oil.

5. Put in hot oven AirFryer and cook for fifteen min at 400° F, spinning the fish halfway around.

6. Divide and serve between plates.

Enjoy it!

Nutrition: 261, Fat: 7 g, Fiber: 18 g, Carbohydrates: 28 g, Protein: 18 g.

13. Seasoned Salmon

Prep Time about 1hr 6 min | Normal

INGREDIENTS:

- ➢ 1 full salmon
- ➢ 1 tablespoon dill, chopped
- ➢ 1 tablespoon of tarragon, hacked
- ➢ 1 tablespoon of garlic, chopped
- ➢ 2 lemon juice.
- ➢ A tablespoon of black pepper and salt

DIRECTIONS:

1. Combine fish with salt, pepper, and lemon juice in a big bowl, shake well, and stir well. Hold in the refrigerator for 1 hour.

2. Stuff salmon with slices of garlic and ginger, place in the basket of your AirFryer. Cook for 25 minutes, at 320° F.

3. Divide between bowls and serve side by side with a wonderful coleslaw.

Enjoy!

Nutrition: Calories: 300, Fat: 8 g, Fiber: 9 g, Carbohydrates: 19 g, Protein: 27 g.

14. Spanish Salmon

Prep Time about 25 min | Servings 6 | Normal

INGREDIENTS:

- ➢ 2 cups of bread
- ➢ 3 red onions, sliced into intermediate wedges
- ➢ 3/4 cup of olives in green, pitted
- ➢ 3 red peppers, sliced into medium-sized wedges
- ➢ 1/2 smoked paprika teaspoon
- ➢ Salt and black chili, to taste
- ➢ 5 lbs of olive oil
- ➢ 6 fair, skinless and boneless salmon fillets
- ➢ 2 peregrinated spoons, chopped

DIRECTIONS:

1. Comb the bread croutons in a heatproof dish that suits your AirFryer. Add the wedges onions, sprinkled bell pepper, olives, salt, paprika, 3 spoonful olive oil, mix good, bring the fryer in the air, and cook for 7 Minutes 356° F.

2. Cover the salmon with the remaining oil, add vegetables, and cook at 360° F for eight minutes.

3. Split the fish and veggie mixture into bowls, spray with the parsley and serve.

Enjoy!

Nutrition: Calories: 321, Fat: 8 g, Fiber: 14 g, Carbohydrates: 27 g, Protein: 22 g.

15. Unique Lettuce

Prep Time about 35 min | Servings 4 | Normal

INGREDIENTS:

- 1 lb medium beet, cut
- 6 pounds of olive oil
- 1**1/2** kilograms of salmon fillets, skinless and boneless
- Salt and chili to taste
- 1 spoonful of chives, chopped
- 1 spoonful of parsley, chopped
- 1 spoonful of fresh tarragon, chopped
- 3 tablespoons of shallots, hacked
- 1 lemon zest rubbed in one cubit
- 1/4 cup juice of a lemon
- 4 cups of organic vegetables for infants

DIRECTIONS:

1. Mix the beets with 1/2 cubic tablespoon of oil in a bowl and swirl to coat.

2. Sprinkle with salt and pepper, put on a baking sheet. Put in a 450° F oven and bake for 20 minutes.

3. Taking the beets out of the oven, introduce the salmon and scatter with the remaining oil and salt and pepper to blend.

4. Comb chives with parsley and tarragon in a bowl, then spray 1 cubit over the salmon.

5. Again, bring into the oven and bake for 15 minutes.

6. In the meantime, in a boil with lemon peel shallots, flour, chili pepper, mix with the lemon juice and the rest of the herbs, and blend properly.

7. Combine 2 spoonfuls of shallots with mixed greens and toss softly.

8. Remove salmon from the oven, set aside on bowls, add beets and greens. Drizzle the remaining shallot dressing over the side and serve right away.

Enjoy it!

Nutrition: Calories: 312, Fat: 2 g, Fiber: 2 g, Protein: 4 g.

16. Salmon Sauce and Greek Yogurt

Prep Time about 10 min | Servings 2 | Normal

INGREDIENTS:

➢ 2 moderate salmon fillets

➢ 1 tsp of chopped basil

➢ Six slices of Lemon

➢ Marine salt and black chili, to taste

➢ 1 cup of Greek yogurt

➢ 2 teaspoons of curry powder

➢ 1 tablespoon of cayenne chili

➢ 1 clove of garlic, minced

➢ 1/2 teaspoon of cilantro

➢ 1/2 teaspoon of mint

DIRECTIONS:

1. Put each salmon fillet on a parchment paper piece, do 3 splits in each piece, and stuff the basil with them.

2. Season with salt and pepper, add 3 slices of lemon to each fillet, fold parchment, sealing corners, 400° F in the oven, and fry for 20 Minutes.

3. Meanwhile, combine the yogurt and the cayenne pepper in a cup, salt to taste, garlic, curry, cilantro, mint, and whisk well.

4. Move fish to bowls, sprinkle with the yogurt sauce you just prepared top, and serve right away!

Enjoy it!

Nutrition: Calories: 242, Fat: 1 g, Carbohydrates: 3 g, Protein: 3 g.

17. Salmon and Avocado Meal

Prep Time about 30 min | Servings 4 | Normal

INGREDIENTS:

➢ 2 medium fillet salmon

➢ 1/4 cup of butter melted

➢ 4 ounces of sliced champignons

➢ Sea salt and black chili, to taste

➢ 12 half cherry tomatoes,

➢ 2 tsp of olive oil

➢ 8 ounces of spinach, ripped

➢ 1 avocado, scalloped, peeled, and cubed

➢ 1 chopped jalapeno pepper

➢ 5 springs of cilantro, chopped

➢ 2 tablespoons of white vinegar

➢ 1 ounce of feta cheese, melted

DIRECTIONS:

1. Place the salmon on a lined baking dish, brush with melted 2 tablespoons of butter, season with salt and pepper, boil over medium heat for 15 minutes, and maintain warm.

2. In the meantime, fire up a skillet over medium heat with the rest of the butter, stir in the mushrooms, then simmer for a couple of minutes.

3. Place the tomatoes in a cup, add salt, pepper, and 1 cubit of olive oil. Toss to switch.

4. Mix salmon with champignons, salmon, avocado, tomatoes in a salad bowl, except cilantro and jalapeno.

5. Add the remaining oil, vinegar, salt, and pepper, sprinkle with the cheese, and then serve.

Enjoy!

Nutrition: Calories: 235, Fat: 6 g, Fiber: 8 g, Carbohydrates: 19 g, Protein: 5 g.

18. Hawaiian Lettuce

Prep Time about 20 min | Servings 2 | Normal

INGREDIENTS:

> 20 ounces of canned bits of pineapple and its juice
> 1/2 ginger paste, rubbed
> 2 spoonful of garlic powder
> 1 teaspoon of powdered onion
> 1 spoonful of balsamic vinegar
> 2 medium, boneless salmon fillets
> Salt and black chili, to taste

DIRECTIONS:

1. Seasoned salmon with garlic powder, salt, and black onion powder pepper, rub well, switch to an air-fitting heat-proof dish Fryer, add bits of ginger pineapple, then mix gently.

2. Clean the vinegar all over, place the fryer in the air, and bake at 350° F for 10 minutes.

3. Split all into plates and serve.

Enjoy!

Nutrition: Calories: 200, Fat: 8 g, Fiber: 12 g, Carbohydrates: 17 g, Protein: 20 g.

19. Cod and Pearl Onions

Prep Time about 10 min | Servings 2 | Normal

INGREDIENTS:

➢ 14 ounces of pearl onions

➢ 2 medium cod fillets

➢ 1 spoonful of parsley, dried

➢ 1 tsp of dried thyme

➢ Yellow chili, to the taste

➢ 8 ounces of sliced champignons

DIRECTIONS:

1. Put the fish in an air-free heat-resistant bowl, add the onions, parsley, beets, thyme, and black pepper, mix well, drop in your bowl. Heat the AirFryer at 350° F, and heat for 15 minutes.

2. On plates split all, and eat.

Enjoy it!

Nutrition: Calories: 270, Fat: 14 g, Fiber: 8 g, Sugars: 14 g, Protein: 22 g.

20. Chinese Cod

Prep Time about 20 min | Servings 2 | Normal

INGREDIENTS:

➢ 2 medium cod fillets, boneless

➢ 1 tsp peanuts, smashed

➢ 2 spoonful of garlic powder

➢ 1 medium tablespoon of soy sauce

➢ 1/2 ginger paste, rubbed

DIRECTIONS:

1. Place the fish fillets in a heat-proof plate that suits your fryer, add the garlic. Brush soy sauce and ginger, stir well, place the fryer in the air and cook for 10 minutes, at 350° F.

2. Divide the fish into bowls, scatter and put the peanuts on top.

Enjoy!

Nutrition: Calories: 254, Fat: 10 g, Fiber: 11 g, Carbohydrates: 14 g, Protein: 23 g.

21. Marine and Seafish

Prep Time about 25 min | Servings 4 | Normal

INGREDIENTS:

- ➢ 2 red onions, sliced
- ➢ Cooking spray
- ➢ 2 small bulbs with fennel, cored and cut
- ➢ 1/4 cup of toasted and sliced almonds
- ➢ Salt and black chili, to taste
- ➢ 2 and 1/2 kilograms of sea bass
- ➢ 5 fennel seeds
- ➢ 3/4 cup of whole couscous flour, cooked

DIRECTIONS:

1. Add salt and pepper cod, spray with cooking spray, put in an AirFryer, and cook for 10 minutes at 350° F.

2. In the meantime, spray a saucepan with some cooking oil and heat over to medium heat.

3. Add, stir and toast fennel seeds to this pan for 1 minute.

4. Add the onion, garlic, chili pepper, fennel, almond, and couscous, whisk, cook 2-3 minutes, and then split between the dishes.

5. Add fish to the couscous mix, and serve immediately.

Enjoy!

Nutrition: Calories: 354, Fat: 7 g, Fiber: 10 g, Carbohydrates: 20 g, Protein: 30 g.

22. Black Cod and Plum Sauce

Prep Time about 25 min | Servings 2 | Normal

INGREDIENTS:

➤ 1 white egg

➤ 1/2 cup of red quinoa, cooked already

➤ 2 tablespoons of whole wheat flour

➤ 4 teaspoons of lemon juice

➤ 1/2 smoked paprika teaspoon

➤ 1 tablespoon of olive oil

➤ 2 skinless and knobbles medium black cod fillets

➤ 1 red plum, chopped and pitted

➤ 2 raw honey teaspoons

➤ 1/4 teaspoons of black peppercorns

➤ 2 Petersil teaspoons

➤ 1/4 bucket of water

DIRECTIONS:

1. In a cup, add 1 teaspoon of lemon juice and a white egg, flour, and 1/4 paprika with a teaspoon and whisk well.

2. Place the quinoa in a bowl and blend with 1/3 white egg mixture.

3. Put the fish in a dish with the former good egg mixture and toss to switch.

4. Sprinkle the fish in a quinoa combination, cover well, and keep on for 10 minutes.

5. Heat a saucepan over medium heat with 1 teaspoon of oil, add the peppercorns, honey, and prune, bring to a boil and prepare for within 1 minute.

6. Apply the remaining lemon juice, the remaining paprika, and the water well, stir and cook for 5 minutes.

7. Add parsley, whisk, extract heat from sauce, and set aside for now.

8. Place the fish in your AirFryer and cook for 10 minutes at 380° F.

9. Arrange fish on bowls, scatter on top with plum sauce and serve.

Enjoy!

Nutrition: Calories: 324, Fat: 14 g, Fiber: 22 g, Carbohydrates: 27 g, Protein: 22 g.

23. Sun-Dried Tomatoes and Halibut Blend

Prep Time about 20 min | Servings 2 | Normal

INGREDIENTS:

- ➢ 2 medium fillets of halibut
- ➢ 2 cloves of garlic, minced
- ➢ 2 tablespoons of olive oil
- ➢ Salt and black chili, to taste
- ➢ Six sun-dried tomatoes, minced
- ➢ Two little red onions, in slices
- ➢ 1 bulb of fennel, cut
- ➢ 9 black, pitted, and diced olives
- ➢ 4 rosemary fountains, chopped
- ➢ 1/2 teaspoon of red pepper flakes

DIRECTIONS:

1. Dress fish with salt, pepper, garlic, and oil and put in a saucepan that's perfect for your AirFryer.

2. Apply slices of cabbage, tomatoes cured by the sun, fennel, olives, rosemary, sprinkle the pepper flakes, move to the Airfryer, and cook 380° F for 10 minutes.

3. Start serving the slice fish and vegetables on bowls. Enjoy!

Nutrition: Calories: 300, Fat: 12 g, Fiber: 9 g, Carbohydrates: 30 g, Protein: 18 g.

24. Prosciutto and Grilled Cod

Prep Time about 20 min | Servings 4 | Normal

INGREDIENTS:

➤ 1 spoonful of parsley, chopped

➤ 4 filets with medium cod

➤ 1/4 cup of butter

➤ 2 cloves of garlic, minced

➤ 2 tsp of lemon juice

➤ 3 prosciutto spoons, chopped

➤ 1 teaspoon of mustard

➤ 1 shallot, cut

➤ Salt and black chili, to taste

DIRECTIONS:

1. In a bowl, blend butter, garlic, parsley, shallot, lemon and mustard, juice, cinnamon, pepper, prosciutto, and whisk well.

2. Season the fish with salt and pepper, scatter the prosciutto all over. Set in the AirFryer and cook for 10 minutes at 390° F.

3. Serve and enjoy!

Nutrition: Calories: 200, Fat: 4 g, Fiber: 7 g, Carbohydrates: 12 g, Protein: 6 g.

25. Vinaigrette Salmon with Chives

Prep Time about 22 min | Servings 4 | Normal

INGREDIENTS:

➤ 2 dill spoons, chopped

➤ Four salmon fillets, boneless

➤ 2 spoonsful of chives, chopped

➤ 1/3 teaspoons of maple syrup

➤ 1 tablespoon of olive oil

➤ 3 spoonsful of balsamic vinegar

➤ Salt and black chili, to taste

DIRECTIONS:

1. Dress fish with salt and pepper, sprinkle with oil, put in the Airfryer, and cook for 8 minutes, tossing once s, at 350°.

2. Heat up a small pot over medium heat with the vinegar, insert the maple sprinkle with sugar, chives, and dill and stir and roast for three minutes.

3. Divide fish into bowls, then serve vinaigrette with chives on top.

Enjoy!

Nutrition: Calories: 270, Fat: 3 g, Fiber: 13 g, Carbohydrates: 25 g, Protein: 10 g.

26. Stuffed Calamari

Prep Time about 35 min | Servings 4 | Normal

INGREDIENTS:

- ➢ 4 large calamari, split and sliced tentacles, and allocated tubes
- ➢ 2 tablespoons of parsley, chopped
- ➢ 5 ounces of kale, chopped
- ➢ 2 garlic cloves, minced
- ➢ 1 chopped red bell pepper
- ➢ 1 tsp of olive oil
- ➢ 2 ounces of tomato canned puree
- ➢ 1 yellow onion, sliced
- ➢ Salt and black chili, to taste

DIRECTIONS:

1. Preheat a saucepan over medium pressure, incorporate onion and garlic. Cook for 2 minutes to combine and prepare.

2. Insert the pepper bell, the tomato puree, the tentacles of calamari, the spinach, salt, and stir in pepper, cook for 10 minutes, then take off fire. Stir in, and cook for three minutes.

3. Stuff calamari tubes with this combination, place in healthy with toothpicks. Cook the AirFryer for 20 minutes at 360° F.

4. Divide calamari into bowls, scatter with parsley and serve.

Enjoy!

Nutrition: Calories: 322, Fat: 10 g, Fiber: 14 g, Carbs: 14 g, Protein: 22 g.

27. Beaked Salmon

Prep Time about 20 min | Servings 4 | Normal

INGREDIENTS:

➢ 1 cup of chopped pistachios

➢ 4 salmon fillets

➢ 1/4 cup juice of a lemon

➢ 2 cups of honey

➢ 1 teaspoon dill, shredded

➢ Salt and black chili, to taste

➢ 1 tablespoon of mustard

DIRECTIONS:

1. Mix the pistachios in a bowl of mustard, sugar, lemon juice, salt. Whisk black pepper then dill, then sprinkle over salmon.

2. Place the AirFryer in and cook for 10 minutes at 350° F.

3. Divide into plates and serve with a salad.

Enjoy!

Nutrition: Calories: 300, Fat: 17 g, Fiber: 12 g, Carbohydrates: 20 g, Protein: 22 g.

28. Salmon and Sauce with Avocado

Prep Time about 20 min | Servings 4 | Normal

INGREDIENTS:

- ➢ 1 avocado, diced, sliced, and peeled
- ➢ 4 Salmon
- ➢ 1/4 cup of cilantro
- ➢ 1/3 tablespoon of coconut milk
- ➢ 1 tsp of lime juice
- ➢ 1 tsp of lime zest, rubbed
- ➢ 1 teaspoon of ground onion
- ➢ 1 teaspoon of crushed garlic
- ➢ Salt and black chili, to taste

DIRECTIONS:

1. Salmon fillets season with salt, black pepper, and lime zest, rub well, put in the AirFryer, cook for 9 minutes at 350° F.

2. Mix avocado and cilantro, garlic powder, in your mixing bowl, powdered cabbage, lime juice, salt, pepper, and coconut milk, blend well, drizzle the salmon over and serve immediately.

Enjoy!

Nutrition: Calories: 260, Fat: 7 g, Fiber: 20 g, Carbohydrates: 28 g, Protein: 18 g.

29. Lemon and Fish Relish

Prep Time about 40 min | Servings 2 | Normal

INGREDIENTS:

➢ 2 salmon fillets, boneless

➢ Salt and black chili, to taste

➢ 1 tbsp of olive oil

To the delight:

➢ 1 tsp lemon juice

➢ 1 shallot, cut

➢ 1 lemon, diced and cut into wedges

➢ 2 peregrinated spoons, chopped

➢ 1/4 cup Olive oil

DIRECTIONS:

1. Season salmon with salt and pepper, fried with ¼ of oil. Put it in the basket of your AirFryer and cook at 320° F for 20 minutes halfway, tossing the fish.

2. Meanwhile, blend shallot and lemon juice in a cup, a sprinkle of salt and black pepper, and keep on for ten mins.

3. Mix the marinated shallot in a different bowl with the lemon slices, salt, parsley, pepper, and 1/4 cup oil and shake well.

4. Divide salmon into bowls, relish and serve top with citrus.

Enjoy!

Nutrition: Calories: 200, Fat: 3 g, Fiber: 3 g, Carbohydrates: 23 g, Protein: 19 g.

30. Chili Salmon

Prep Time about 25 min | Servings 12 | Normal

INGREDIENTS:

➢ 1 and a half cups of coconut, shredded

➢ 1 lb of salmon, cubed

➢ 1/3 teaspoons of flour

➢ 1 tablespoon of black pepper and salt

➢ 1 egg

➢ 2 tsp of olive oil

➢ 1/4 bowl of water

➢ 4 red chilies, sliced

➢ 3 cloves of garlic, minced

➢ Balsamic vinegar: 1/4 cup

➢ One and a half cup of honey

DIRECTIONS:

1. Place flour and a pinch of salt in a bowl, then whisk.

2. Blend the egg with black pepper and mix it in another bowl.

3. Place the coconut in a separate saucepan.

4. Sprinkle the salmon cubes with flour, egg, and coconut, drop them in your air basket fryer, cook for 8 minutes at 370° F, tossing midway, then divide between plates.

5. Heat up a saucepan with water at medium pressure, add chilies, cloves, honey, and vinegar, stir well, add to boil. Drizzle over salmon for a few moments, then serve.

Enjoy it!

Nutrition: Calories: 220, Fat: 12 g, Fiber: 2 g, Carbohydrates: 14 g, Protein: 13 g.

31. Marmalade of Savory and Orange

Prep Time about 25 min | Servings 4 | Normal

INGREDIENTS:

➢ 1 lb of wild salmon, skinless, ossified, and cubed

➢ 2 cut lemons

➢ 1/4 cup Balsamic vinegar

➢ 1/4 tablespoon of orange juice

➢ 1/3 tablespoon of orange marmalade

➢ A tablespoon of black pepper and salt

DIRECTIONS:

1. Heat the vinegar in a pot over medium pressure, add marmalade, and the orange juice, stir, simmer for 1 minute and bring to a boil. Let it off.

2. Cut salmon and slices of lemon on skewers, season with salt, rub them with half the orange marmalade and black pepper. Mix, put in the basket of your AirFryer, and cook at 360 F for 3 minutes.

3. Pinch skewers with the majority of the vinegar mixture, divided between, cover with a side salad, and serve promptly.

Enjoy!

Nutrition: Calories: 240, Fat: 9 g, Fiber: 12 g, Carbohydrates: 14 g, Protein: 10 g.

32. Swordfish, with Salsa Mango

Prep Time about 16 min | Servings 2 | Normal

INGREDIENTS:

- ➢ 2 medium steaks with swordfish
- ➢ Salt and black chili, to taste
- ➢ 2 tsp of avocado oil
- ➢ 1 spoonful of cilantro, chopped
- ➢ 1 mango, split
- ➢ 1 avocado, diced, sliced, and peeled
- ➢ A clump of cumin
- ➢ A pinch of onion powder
- ➢ A small bit of garlic powder
- ➢ 1 lime, cut and peeled
- ➢ 1/2 cubic of balsamic vinegar

DIRECTIONS:

1. Fish steaks season with salt, vinegar, garlic powder, onion powder, and apply half of the oil to the cumin and clean, put in the AirFryer and cook for 6 minutes at 360° F, turning in half.

2. Meanwhile, blend avocado and mango in a bowl, cilantro, and balsamic vinegar, salt, pepper, and remaining oil, mix well.

3. Splash the cod, fill with mango salsa and serve with orange slices sideways.

Enjoy!

Nutrition: Calories: 200, Fat: 7 g, Fiber: 2 g, Carbohydrates: 14 g, Protein: 14 g.

33. Thai Fish Cakes AirFryer Style

Prep Time about 35 min | Servings 4 | Normal

INGREDIENTS:

➢ 1 cup of potatoes, mashed

➢ 2 cups of white fish

➢ 1 small onion

➢ 1 tsp of butter

➢ 1 tsp of milk

➢ 1 (zest and rind) lime

➢ 3 chili tsp

➢ 1 tsp of Worcester sauce

➢ 1 tsp of coriander

➢ 1 tsp of blended wheat

➢ 1 tsp of mixed herbs

➢ Breadcrumbs (from 1 slice of bread)

➢ Salt and pepper to the taste

DIRECTIONS:

1. Place the fish white in a wide saucepan and cover with milk.

2. Put a large mixing bowl with the drained poached cod. Put the seasoning on mash potatoes, and blend properly. Mash well before lumps-free.

3. Apply the butter and milk and whisk well.

4. Shape into fish cakes and cool for 3 hours.

5. Cook on 200° F heat in AirFryer for fifteen minutes.

Nutrition: Calories: 221, Fat: 2 g, Protein: 4 g.

34. Aromatized Jamaican Salmon

Prep Time about 20 min | Servings 4 | Normal

INGREDIENTS:

➢ 2 sriracha sauce with teaspoons

➢ 4 sugar teaspoons

➢ 3 chopped scallions

➢ Salt and black chili, to taste

➢ 2 tablespoons of olive oil

➢ 4 tablespoons cider apple vinegar

➢ 3 pockets of avocado oil

➢ 4 medium-size fillets of salmon, boneless

➢ 4 cups of arugula

➢ 2 cups of fish, shredded

➢ 1 and 1/2 teaspoon of seasoning Jamaican jerk

➢ 1/4 cup of toasted pepitas

➢ 2 radish tassels, julienned

DIRECTIONS:

1. Mix the sriracha and sugar in a cup, whisk, and move.

2. Mix 2 spoonsful of sriracha with avocado oil, olive oil, vinegar, pepper, and salt and shake well.

3. Sprinkle with salmon seasoning, bake with sriracha and sugar. Mix with salt and pepper, then season.

4. Switch to the AirFryer and cook for 10 minutes at 360° F, one tossing.

5. Mix radishes in a bowl of diced chicken, rye, salt, pepper, vinegar, and sriracha combined and thrown together.

6. Splash the salmon and radish into bowls, add the pepitas and top scallions and eat.

Enjoy!

Nutrition: Calories: 290, Fat: 6g, Fiber: 12g, Carbohydrates: 17g, Protein: 10g.

35. Mustard Salmon

Prep Time about 20 min | Servings 1 | Normal

INGREDIENTS:

➢ 1 big, boneless salmon fillet

➢ Salt and black chili, to taste

➢ Two mustard spoons

➢ 1 tsp of coconut oil

➢ 1 tablespoon of maple

DIRECTIONS:

1. Mix the maple extract and mustard in a bowl, whisk well, season well the salmon with salt and pepper, and salmon brown with this combination.

2. Sprinkle some cooking spray over fish, put it in the AirFryer, and cook 10 minutes at 370° F, turning in half.

3. Serve with a flavorful salad on the side.

Enjoy!

Nutrition: Calories: 300, Fat: 7g, Fiber: 14g, Carbohydrates: 16g, Protein: 20g.

36. Flaked Salmon

Prep Time about 30 min | Servings 2 | Normal

INGREDIENTS:

- ➢ 2 salmon fillets, skinless and without bones
- ➢ 1 tablespoon of olive oil
- ➢ 5 ounces of tiger shrimp, roasted, sliced, and deveined
- ➢ 6 champignons, split
- ➢ 3 cut green onions,
- ➢ 2 cups spinach, ripped apart
- ➢ 1/4 cup of macadamia nuts, toasted and chopped
- ➢ Salt and black chili, to taste

DIRECTIONS:

1. Heat one saucepan with half the oil over medium pressure, insert mushrooms, tomatoes, salt, and pepper, and whisk and cook for 4 minutes.

2. Include macadamia spinach and shrimp, whisk, simmer for 3 minutes, and take the heat off.

3. Incision the salmon fillet lengthwise, season with salt, and mustard, spinach, and shrimp blend together incisions and rub olive oil, with the remainder.

4. Put in the basket of your AirFryer and cook at 360° F, flipping midway, for 10 minutes.

5. Divide and serve stewed salmon on bowls.

Enjoy!

Nutrition: Calories: 290, Fat: 3g, Fiber: 15g, Carbohydrates: 12g, Protein: 31g.

37. Shrimp and Cauliflower

Prep Time about 22 min | Servings 2 | Normal

INGREDIENTS:

➢ 1 tablespoon of butter

➢ Cooking spray

➢ 1 head of cauliflower, riced

➢ 1 pound of shrimps, sliced

➢ 1/4 cup of milk

➢ 8 ounces of champignons, sliced roughly

➢ 1 tablespoon of red potato flakes

➢ Salt and black chili, to taste

➢ 2 cloves of garlic, minced

➢ 4 slices of bacon, fried and sliced

➢ 1/2 cup of beef

➢ 1 spoonful of parsley, finely chopped

➢ 1 spoonful of chives, chopped

DIRECTIONS:

1. Add salt and pepper shrimp, spray with cooking oil, put in an AirFryer, and cook for 7 minutes at 360° F.

2. In the meantime, prepare a saucepan over medium heat with butter, add stir in the mushrooms, and simmer for 3-4 minutes.

3. Add garlic, rice of cauliflower, flakes of pepper, stock, cream, peppers, stir in parsley, salt, and pepper, simmer for a few minutes, then take off the heat.

4. Break the shrimp into bowls, apply the cauliflower mixture on the side, sprinkle bacon, and serve.

Enjoy it!

Nutrition: Calories: 245, Fat: 7g, Fiber: 4g, Carbohydrates: 6g, Protein: 20g.

38. Squid and Guacamole

Prep Time about 16 min | Servings 2 | Normal

INGREDIENTS:

➢ 2 medium squids, distinct tentacles, and graded longitudinally

➢ 1 tablespoon of olive oil

➢ 1 lime Juice

➢ Salt and black chili, to taste

For the guacamole:

➢ 2 avocados, pitted, sliced, and peeled

➢ 1 tsp, chopped coriander

➢ 2 red chilies, sliced

➢ 1 tomato, sliced

➢ 1 red onion, sliced

➢ 2 lemon juice

DIRECTIONS:

1. Sprinkle the olive with lemon, vinegar, squid, and squid tentacles. Put oil in your AirFryer basket and cook 360° F at either size for 3 minutes.

2. Switch squid to a bowl, drizzle, and sprinkle lime juice all over.

3. In the meanwhile, place the avocado in a cup, mash with a fork, add chilies, coriander, peppers, onion, and 2 lime juice, then shake.

4. Divide squid into bowls, cover, and serve with guacamole.

Enjoy!

Nutrition: Calories: 500, weight 43g, Fiber: 6g, Carbohydrates: 7g, Protein: 20g.

39. Chimichurri and Fish Sauce

Prep Time about 18 min | Servings 4 | Normal

INGREDIENTS:

➢ 1/2 cup cilantro, sliced

➢ 1/3 cup of olive oil + 2 spoonful

➢ 1 small, chopped red onion

➢ 3 1/2 cubit of balsamic vinegar

➢ 2 tsp of parsley, chopped

➢ 2 cubits of basil, minced

➢ 1 chopped jalapeno pepper

➢ 1 pound of steak with spicy tuna

➢ Salt and black chili, to taste

➢ 1 teaspoon of red flakes

➢ 1 teaspoon of thyme, cut

➢ 3 cloves of garlic, minced

➢ 2 avocados, bruised, sliced, and peeled

➢ 6 ounces of arugula

DIRECTIONS:

1. Mix 1/3 of the oil in a bowl with the jalapeno, vinegar, cabbage, cilantro, basil, ginger, parsley, thyme, salt, and pepper spray, whisk well, and now put aside.

2. Season the tuna with salt and pepper, fried the remaining oil, put in the fryer, and cook for 3 minutes at 360° F on each side.

3. Combine the arugula with half the chimichurri blend and throw to flirt with.

4. Break the arugula into bowls, dice the tuna, split into them, top chimichurri with the remainder, and eat.

Enjoy!

Nutrition: Calories: 276, Fat: 3g, Fiber: 1g, Carbohydrates: 14g, Protein: 20g.

40. Creamy Vegetables and Shrimp

Prep Time about 40 min | Servings 4 | Normal

INGREDIENTS:

➢ 8 ounces of champignons, chopped

➢ 1 bunch of asparagus, sliced into medium bits

➢ 1 pound Shrimp, peeled

➢ Salt and black chili, to taste

➢ 1 spaghetti squash, half-cut

➢ 2 oz of olive oil

➢ 2 teaspoons Italian seasoning

➢ 1 yellow onion, sliced

➢ 1 teaspoon of red, crushed pepper flakes

➢ 1/4 cup of butter, molten,

➢ 1 cup of parmesan cheese

➢ 2 cloves of garlic, minced

➢ 1 cup of heavy cream

DIRECTIONS:

1. Place half of the squash in the fryer's basket, cook 390° F for 17 minutes. Transfer to the cutting board, scoop insides and switch to the bowl.

2. Put water in a saucepan, add some iodine, boil over medium heat, add asparagus, steam, and switch to a bowl for a few minutes. Loaded with ice water, then drain and set aside.

3. Heat a pan that matches the oil to your AirFryer over medium pressure, add the mushrooms and onions, and stir and simmer for 7 minutes.

4. Connect the pepper flakes, milk, vinegar, onion, Italian seasoning, toss asparagus, lobster, butter melted, cheese, parmesan, and garlic, and bake in an AirFryer for 6 minutes at 360 ° Fahrenheit.

5. On plates, divide all and serve.

Enjoy it!

Nutrition: Calories: 325, Fat: 6g, Fiber: g 5, Carbohydrates: 14g, Protein: 13g.

41. Italian Tomato Salsa and Barramundi Filets

Prep Time about 18 min | Servings 4 | Normal

INGREDIENTS:

- ➢ 2 barramundi, boneless filets
- ➢ One tablespoon of olive oil + 2 teaspoons
- ➢ Two teaspoons Italian seasoning
- ➢ 1/4 cup of green olives, diced and pitted
- ➢ 1/4 cup Cherry tomatoes, chopped
- ➢ 1/4 cup of black olives
- ➢ 1 cubic lemon zest
- ➢ 2 lemon zest spoons
- ➢ Salt and black chili, to taste
- ➢ 2 tsp parsley, chopped

DIRECTIONS:

1. Add salt, pepper, Italian seasoning, and 2 teaspoons of olive oil. Transfer the oil to your AirFryer and cook for 8 minutes at 360° F, halfway, tossing them.

2. Mix the tomatoes in a dish with black olives, green olives, salt, pepper, lemon zest, lemon juice, parsley, and 1 tbs of olive oil. Toss well.

3. Divide the fish into bowls, fill with tomato salsa and eat.

Enjoy!

Nutrition: Calories: 270, Fat: 4g, Fiber: 2g, Carbohydrates: 18g, Protein: 27g.

42. Salsa with Salmon and Avocado

Prep Time about 40 min | Servings 4 | Normal

INGREDIENTS:

- ➢ 4 salmon fillets
- ➢ 1 tablespoon of olive oil
- ➢ Salt and black chili, to taste
- ➢ 1 tsp of ground cumin
- ➢ 1 litter of tender paprika
- ➢ 1/2 cup of chili powder
- ➢ 1 teaspoon of crushed garlic

For the salsa:

- ➢ 1 thin, chopped red onion
- ➢ 1 avocado, diced, sliced, and peeled
- ➢ 2 cilantro teaspoons, chopped
- ➢ 2 lemon juice
- ➢ Salt and black chili, to taste

DIRECTIONS:

1. In a cup, add flour, chili powder, pepper, onion powder, paprika, and cumin, whisk, scrape the salmon with this combination, cut the grease, scrape again. Switch to your fryer, and cook for 5 mins at 350° F on each side.

2. In the meantime, blend the avocado with red onion, salt, pepper in a cup, stir and add cilantro and lime juice.

3. Divide fillets into bowls, cover with salsa and serve with avocado.

Enjoy!

Nutrition: Calories: 300, Fat: 14g, Fiber: 4g, Carbohydrates: 18g, Protein: 16g.

43. Creamy Salmon

Prep Time about 20 min | Servings 4 | Normal

INGREDIENTS:

➢ 4 salmon fillets, boneless

➢ 1 spoonful of olive oil

➢ Salt and black chili, to taste

➢ 1/3 cup of cheddar cheese, brushed together

➢ 1 and a half teaspoon of mustard

➢ 1/2 cup of milk coconut

DIRECTIONS:

1. Season salmon with salt and pepper, cut the oil and rinse well.

2. In a bowl, add the cheddar, mustard, salt, and coconut cream, pepper, and mix well.

3. Move salmon into a saucepan that suits your fryer and add coconut cream, mix, put in the AirFryer, and cook for 10 minutes at 320° F.

4. Divide between plates and eat.

Enjoy!

Nutrition: Calories: 200, Fat: 6g, Fiber: 14g, Carbohydrates: 17g Protein: 20g.

44. Trout and Sauce with Butter

Prep Time about 20 min | Servings 4 | Normal

INGREDIENTS:

- ➤ 4 fillets of trout boneless
- ➤ Salt and black chili, to taste
- ➤ 3 lemon zest spoons rubbed
- ➤ 3 spoonsful of chives, chopped
- ➤ 6 tablespoons of butter
- ➤ 2 tablespoons of olive oil
- ➤ 2 teaspoons of lemon juice

DIRECTIONS:

1. Season with salt and pepper, drizzle with olive oil, bake, move to the AirFryer and cook for 10 minutes at 360° F.

2. In the meantime, prepare a saucepan over medium heat with butter, add salt, vinegar, vinegar, lemon juice, and zest, whisk well, boil 1-2 minutes and take off the heat.

3. Split fish fillets into bowls, add butter sauce and serve all over.

Enjoy!

Nutrition: Calories: 300, Fat: 12g, Fiber: 9g, Carbohydrates: 27g, Protein: 24g.

45. Thyme and Parsley Salmon

Prep Time about 25 min | Servings 4 | Normal

INGREDIENTS:

➢ 4 salmon fillets boneless

➢ 1 lemon juice

➢ 1 yellow onion, sliced

➢ 3 tomatoes, diced

➢ 4 thyme fountains

➢ 4 springs of parsley

➢ 3 spoonfuls of extra virgin olive oil

➢ Salt and black chili, to taste

DIRECTIONS:

1. Sprinkle 1 spoonful of oil in a saucepan that suits your AirFryer, add tomatoes, salt, and chili pepper, add 1 more spoonful of oil, water, sauté them with salt and pepper, sprinkle the remaining oil. Add springs of thyme and parsley, mushrooms, lemon juice, lime, and spice pepper, put in the basket of your AirFryer, and cook 360° F for 12 minutes.

2. On plates, split all and serve immediately.

Enjoy!

Nutrition: Calories: 242, Fat: 9g, Fiber: 12g, Carbohydrates: 20g, Protein: 31g.

46. Fillet Cod and Peas

Prep Time about 20 min | Servings 4 | Normal

INGREDIENTS:

- ➢ 4 cod fillets, boneless
- ➢ 2 tablespoons of parsley, chopped
- ➢ 2 cups of peas
- ➢ 4 tablespoons of wine
- ➢ 2 tsp of oregano, dry
- ➢ 1/2 cup of tender paprika
- ➢ 2 cloves of garlic, minced
- ➢ Salt and chili to taste

DIRECTIONS:

1. Mix the garlic with the parsley, salt, pepper in your mixing bowl, add oregano, paprika, and juice, mix well.

2. Rub the fish with half of this combination, put in the air fryer, and cook for 10 minutes at 360° F.

3. In the meantime, place the peas in a kettle, add water to cover, add salt and bring to boil over medium pressure, simmer for ten minutes. Divide into plates.

4. Divide fish into bowls, scatter the rest of the herb dressing over and serve.

Enjoy it!

Nutrition: Calories: 261, Fat: 8g, Fiber: 12g, Carbohydrates: 20g, Protein: 22g.

47. Fillet Truffle and Orange Sauce

Prep Time about 20 min | Servings 4 | Normal

INGREDIENTS:

➢ 4 fillets of trout, skinless and boneless

➢ 4 onions in the spring, minced

➢ 1 tablespoon of olive oil

➢ 1 tablespoon of ginger, minced

➢ Salt and black chili, to taste

➢ 1 orange juice and zest

DIRECTIONS:

1. Season the fillets with salt and pepper, rub them with the oil, put them in a saucepan that suits your fryer, add the ginger, the green onions, orange zest, and juice, stir well, place in the fryer, and cook for 10 minutes at 360° F.

2. Divide fish and sauce into bowls and serve immediately.

Enjoy!

Nutrition: Calories: 239, Fat: 10g, Fiber: 7g, Carbohydrates: 18g, Protein: 23g.

48. Casserole Seafood

Prep Time about 50 min | Servings 6 | Normal

INGREDIENTS:

- ➤ 6 tablespoons of butter
- ➤ 2 ounces of champignons, chopped
- ➤ 1 little green bell pepper chopped
- ➤ 1 stalk of celery hacked
- ➤ 2 cloves of garlic, minced
- ➤ 1 small yellow, diced onion
- ➤ Salt and black chili, to taste
- ➤ 4 teaspoons of flour
- ➤ 1/2 cup White wine
- ➤ 1 and a half cups of milk
- ➤ 4 Scallops at sea, cut
- ➤ 4 ounces of haddock, skinless, boneless and cut into small parts
- ➤ 4 ounces of lobster meat already cooked and cut into small pieces
- ➤ 1/2 teaspoon of mustard powder
- ➤ 1 tablespoon of lemon juice
- ➤ 1/3 cup of crumbs of bread
- ➤ Salt and black chili, to taste
- ➤ 3 spoonfuls of cheddar cheese, grated
- ➤ 1 tablespoon of sliced parsley

➢ 1 teaspoon of sweet paprika

DIRECTIONS:

1. Heat a saucepan with 4 spoons of butter over medium pressure, whisk in bell pepper, chestnuts, celery, garlic, onion, and wine. Then, boil for ten minutes.

2. Stir well and simmer for 6 minutes. Add flour, cream, and milk.

3. Add lemon juice, salt, pepper, ground mustard, scallops, lobster, meat, and haddock, stir well, heat off, and transfer to a saucepan that fits the fryer.

4. Mix the remaining butter in a dish with the breadcrumbs, paprika, and sprinkle with cheese over the seafood mixture.

5. Switch the saucepan to the AirFryer and cook at 360° F for 16 minutes.

6. Divide between bowls, then serve sprinkled on top of parsley.

Enjoy!

Nutrition: Calories: 270, Fat: 32g, Fiber: 14g, Carbohydrates: 15g, Protein: 23g.

49. Shrimp and Mix with Crab

Prep Time about 35 min | Servings 4 | Normal

INGREDIENTS:

- ➤ 1/2 cup of yellow, minced onion
- ➤ 1 cup of green potatoes, diced
- ➤ 1 cup of celery, cut
- ➤ 1 pound of crawls, sliced
- ➤ 1 cup of crabmeat, sliced
- ➤ 1 cup of mayonnaise
- ➤ 1 teaspoon Worcestershire sauce
- ➤ Salt and black chili, to taste
- ➤ 2 sliced of bread
- ➤ 1 tablespoon of butter, melted
- ➤ 1 tablespoon of tender paprika

DIRECTIONS:

1. Combine shrimp and crab meat in a dish, bell pepper, tomato, mayo, sauce with celery, garlic, chili pepper, and Worcestershire, mix well and pass to the casserole that suits your fryer.

2. Sprinkle the crumbs and the paprika with the crust, apply the melted butter, and put in your AirFryer and bake for 25 minutes at 320° F, midway.

3. Divide between bowls and serve immediately.

Enjoy!

Nutrition: Calories: 200, Fat: 13g, Fiber: 9g, Carbohydrates: 17g, Protein: 19g.

50. Cod and Vinaigrette

Prep Time about 25 min | Servings 4 | Normal

INGREDIENTS:

➢ 4 cod fillets, skinless and boneless

➢ 12 halved cherry tomatoes

➢ 8 black olives, finely chopped and pitted

➢ 2 tablespoons of lemon juice

➢ Salt and black chili, to taste

➢ 2 tablespoons of olive oil

➢ Cooking spray

➢ 1 packet of basil, chopped

DIRECTIONS:

1. Season cod with salt and pepper to taste, put in the AirFryers bucket, and cook for 10 minutes at 360° F for five minutes.

2. In the meantime, prepare a saucepan over medium heat with the oil, add the onions, olives, and lemon juice, bring to a boil, add basil. Stir well with salt and pepper, and take off fire.

3. Segregate fish into plates and serve on top with the drizzled vinaigrette.

Enjoy!

Nutrition: Calories: 300, Fat: 5g, Fiber: 8g, Carbohydrates: 12g, Protein: 8g.

51. Asian Halibut

Prep Time about 40 min | Servings 3 | Normal

INGREDIENTS:

- ➢ 1 lb. of halibut steaks
- ➢ 2/3 cup Soy sauce
- ➢ 1 and a half cup of sugar
- ➢ 2 spoonful of lime juice
- ➢ 1/2 cup of mirin
- ➢ 1/4 teaspoon red pepper flakes
- ➢ 1/4 tablespoon of orange juice
- ➢ 1/4 tablespoon of ginger powder, grated
- ➢ 1 clove of garlic, minced

DIRECTIONS:

1. Place soy sauce in a saucepan, heat over a moderate flame, including mirin, sugar, lime and orange juice, ginger and garlic, pepper flakes, mix well. Bring it to a boil, and heat off.

2. Put half of the marinade in a bowl, add halibut, toss to cover, then leave them in the refrigerator for 30 minutes.

3. Switch the halibut to the AirFryer and cook for 10 minutes at 390° F, only flipping once.

4. Divide halibut steaks into bowls, scatter with the rest of the marinade. Serve and enjoy!

Nutrition: Calories: 286, Fat: 5g, Fiber: 12g, Carbohydrates: 14g, Protein: 23g.

52. Marine Lemon Saba

Prep Time about 18 min | Servings 1 | Normal

INGREDIENTS:

➢ 4 Sheba fish fillets

➢ Salt and black chili, to taste

➢ 3 red peppered chilies, minced

➢ 2 tablespoons of lemon juice

➢ 2 1/2 cubit of olive oil

➢ 2 teaspoons of garlic, chopped

DIRECTIONS:

1. Season fish fillets and place them in a bowl of salt and pepper.

2. Add lemon juice, milk, chili, and garlic to coat, and pass to the freezer the air and cook for 8 minutes at 360° F, midway.

3. Divide between bowls and serve with a few fries.

Enjoy it!

Nutrition: Calories: 300, Fat: 4g, Fiber: 8g, Carbohydrates: 15g, Protein: 15g.

53. Salmon with Capers and Mash

Prep Time about 30 min | Servings 4 | Normal

INGREDIENTS:

- ➢ 4 skinless and boneless salmon fillets
- ➢ 1 spoonful of caper, drained
- ➢ Salt and black chili, to taste
- ➢ 1 lemon juice
- ➢ 2 cups of olive oil

For mash potatoes:

- ➢ 2 tablespoons of olive oil
- ➢ 1 tablespoon of dill, dry
- ➢ 1 pound of diced potatoes
- ➢ 1/2 cup of milk

DIRECTIONS:

1. Place the potatoes in a saucepan, add a little water, add some salt, bring to boil over a moderate flame, cook for fifteen min, drain, switch to low heat. In a bowl, pound with a potato masher, add 2 cubic cubes of oil, dill, honey, and whisk the pepper and milk good, and set aside for now.

2. Season salmon with salt and pepper and drizzle 2 teaspoons oil over them, rub, and transfer to the basket of your AirFryer, add capers on top. Cook for 8 minutes, at 360° F.

3. Break salmon and capers into bowls, add mashed potatoes to the pan, drizzle the lemon juice over **the** side and eat.

Enjoy!

Nutrition: Calories: 300, Fat: 17g, Fiber: 8g, Carbohydrates: 12g, Protein: 18g.

54. Aromatized Air Fried Salmon

Prep Time about 1hr 8 min | Servings 2 | Normal

INGREDIENTS:

- ➤ 2 salmon fillets
- ➤ 2 tablespoons of lemon juice
- ➤ Salt and black chili, to taste
- ➤ 1/2 teaspoon crushed garlic
- ➤ 1/3 cup of soy sauce
- ➤ 3 chopped scallions
- ➤ 1/3 cup of brown sugar
- ➤ 2 tablespoons of olive oil

DIRECTIONS:

1. In a bowl, add water to the sugar, soy sauce, garlic powder, salt. Sprinkle with oil, and lemon juice, whisk well, add salmon fillets and toss. Cover in the fridge and set aside for 1 hour.

2. Move the salmon fillets into the basket of the fryer and cook at 360° F, flipping them in half for 8 minutes.

3. Divide the salmon into bowls, scatter the scallions on top and serve appropriately.

Enjoy it!

Nutrition: Calories: 300, Fat: 12g, Fiber: 10g, Carbohydrates: 23g, Protein: 20g.

55. Steaks Cod with Plum Sauce

Prep Time about 30 min | Servings 2 | Normal

INGREDIENTS:

➢ 2 big cod steaks

➢ Salt and black chili, to taste

➢ 1/2 teaspoon crushed garlic

➢ 1/2 cubicle ginger powder

➢ 1/4 tablespoon of turmeric powder

➢ 1 tablespoon of plum sauce

➢ Cooking spray

DIRECTIONS:

1. Season cod steaks with salt and pepper, sprinkle with cream, apply powdered garlic, ginger powder, and turmeric powder, and rub well.

2. Place cod steaks in your AirFryer and cook for 15 Minutes at 360° F, after 7 minutes.

3. Heat a casserole over medium heat, add prune sauce, stir and cook for just 2 minutes.

4. Divide the cod steaks into bowls, drizzle all over the plum sauce and serve.

Enjoy!

Nutrition: Calories: 250; Fat: 7, Fiber: 1, 14 Carbohydrates, 12g Protein: 24g

56. Asian Salmon

Prep Time about 1hr 15 min | Servings 2 | Normal

INGREDIENTS:

➢ 2 moderate fillet salmon

➢ 6 spoonsful of medium soy sauce

➢ Three teaspoons mirin

➢ 1 tablespoon of water

➢ Six spoons honey

DIRECTIONS:

1. Mix the soy sauce and honey, water, and mirin in a container, shake well. Bring salmon, rub well, and put in the refrigerator for 1 hour.

2. Transfer the salmon to the AirFryer and cook for 15 minutes, at 360° F; after 7 minutes, flip.

3. Put the soy marinade in a saucepan, flame over medium heat up, whisk properly, simmer for 2 minutes, and turn off.

4. Break salmon on bowls, chop marinade all over, and eat.

Enjoy!

Nutrition: Calories: 300, Fat: 12g, Fiber: 8g, Carbohydrates: 13g, Protein: 24g.

57. Buttered Shrimp Skewers

Prep Time about 16 min | Servings 2 | Normal

INGREDIENTS:

➢ 8 shrimps, sliced

➢ 4 cloves of garlic, diced

➢ Salt and black chili, to taste

➢ 8 slices of green bell pepper

➢ 1 spoonful of rosemary, chopped

➢ 1 tablespoon of butter, melted

DIRECTIONS:

1. Mix the shrimp with the garlic, butter, salt, pepper, rosemary in a dish, and slices of pepper bell, swirl to cover, and keep on for ten minutes.

2. Put 2 shrimp and 2 slices of bell pepper on a skewer and repeat for the remaining bits of shrimp and bell pepper.

3. Place all in the basket of your AirFryer and cook 360° F for six minutes.

4. Separate between bowls, and serve immediately.

Enjoy!

Nutrition: Calories: 140, Fat: 1g, Fiber: 12g, Carbohydrates: 15g, Protein: 7g.

58. Shrimp Tabasco

Prep Time about 20 min | Servings 4 | Normal

INGREDIENTS:

➢ 1 pound of shrimps, sliced

➢ 1 teaspoon red pepper flakes

➢ 2 tablespoons of olive oil

➢ 1 Tabasco teaspoon sauce

➢ 2 cups of water

➢ 1 tsp of dried oregano

➢ Salt and black chili, to taste

➢ 1/2 teaspoon of dried parsley

➢ 1/2 smoked paprika teaspoon

DIRECTIONS:

1. Mix oil and water in a bowl, Tabasco sauce, pepper flakes, oregano, parsley, rice, vinegar, bell pepper, shrimp, and mix well.

2. Transfer shrimps to 370° F to your hot oven AirFryer and cook, turning the fryer once for ten minutes.

3. On bowls, split the shrimp and serve with a side salad.

Enjoy it!

Nutrition: Calories: 200, Fat: 6g, Fiber: 13g, Carbohydrates: 8g, Protein: 46g

59. Cod Cutlets with Salad Fennel and Grapes

Prep Time about 25 min | Servings 2 | Normal

INGREDIENTS:

- ➤ 2 fillets of black cod, boneless
- ➤ 1 tablespoon of olive oil
- ➤ Salt and black chili, to taste
- ➤ 1 bulb of fennel, thinly sliced
- ➤ 1 cup of grapes
- ➤ 1/2 cup of pecans

DIRECTIONS:

1. Put half of the oil to the fillets, season with salt and pepper, scrub well, put fillets in the basket of your AirFryer, and cook for 10 minutes at 400° F and transfer to a plate.

2. Combine pecans in a bowl with grapes, fennel, residual oil, salt, and pepper, stir in the coat, add to the saucepan, which suits your fryer, and cook for five minutes, at 400° Fahrenheit.

3. Split the cod into bowls, add the fennel and the pecans on the side, and serve.

Enjoy it!

Nutrition: Calories: 300g, Fat: 4g, Fiber: 2g, Carbohydrates: 32g, Protein: 22g.

60. Tasty Catfish

Prep Time about 30 min | Servings 4 | Normal

INGREDIENTS:

➢ 4 fillets of catfish

➢ Salt and black chili, to taste

➢ A small pinch of sweet paprika

➢ 1 spoonful of parsley, diced

➢ 1 tablespoon of lemon juice

➢ 1 tablespoon of olive oil

DIRECTIONS:

1. Catfish fillets coat with salt, pepper, paprika, grease, rub well, put in the AirFryer basket, and cook for 20 minutes at 400° F, after 10 minutes. The fish must be rotated.

2. Divide fish between bowls, sprinkle with lemon juice, sprinkle with parsley, and serve

Enjoy!

Nutrition: Calories: 253, Fat: 6g, Fiber: 12g, Carbohydrates: 26g, Protein: 22g.

Lightning Source UK Ltd.
Milton Keynes UK
UKHW020641270521
384471UK00010B/758